SUICIDAL THOUGHTS

How to Reduce Suicidal Thoughts and Tendencies

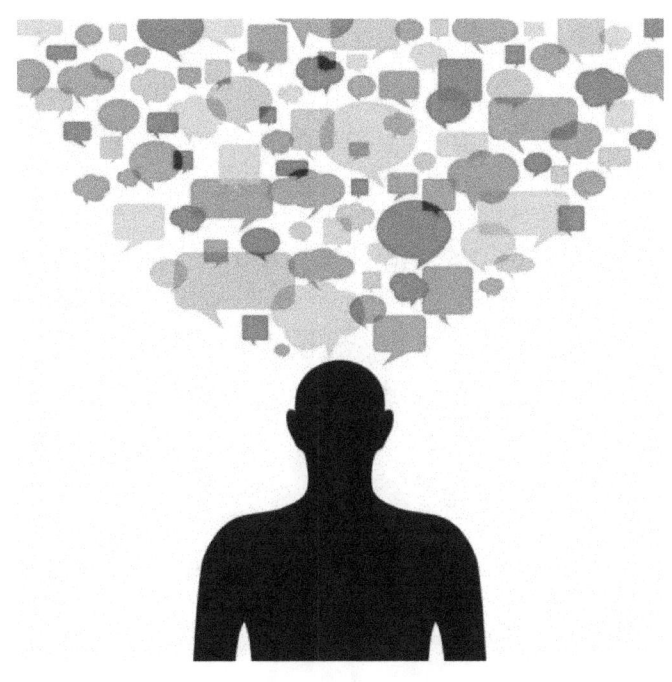

By Patricia A. Carlisle

Introduction

I want to thank you and congratulate you for choosing the book, *"SUICIDAL THOUGHTS: How to Reduce Suicidal Thoughts and Tendencies"*.

This book contains proven steps and strategies on what you should do if you are having suicidal thoughts.

Suicidal thoughts can quickly lead to tragedies, and you need to know how to help yourself. In order to do something about your thoughts, you should learn how to cope with your hurts, grief, or pain and overcome it.

Most of the time a person going through the feeling of having nothing to live for will not share his or her suicidal thoughts with anyone. In this case it can be harder to get help, but not impossible. Suicidal thoughts must be taken seriously. It is important to do all you can to overcome your feelings of despair.

Thanks again for choosing this book, I hope you enjoy it!

TABLE OF CONTENT

Chapter 9

GO TO THERAPY

Preview Of 'THE DEPRESSION CURE: How to Overcome Depression and become Depression Free'

Chapter 1

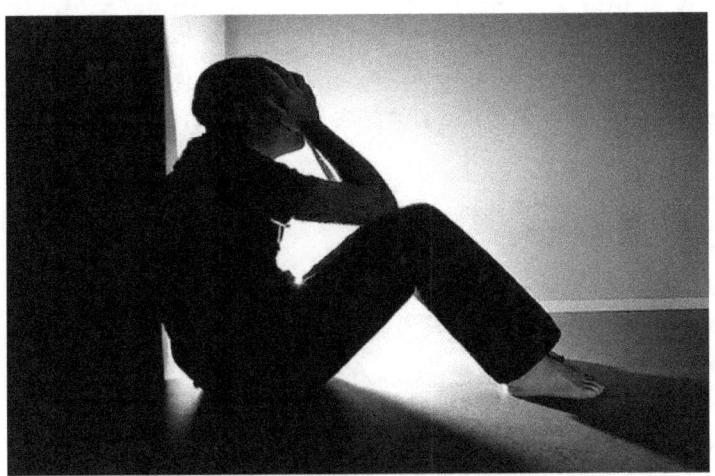

GET TREATMENT FOR YOUR DEPRESSION

Depression is closely linked to suicidal thoughts. This is why you need to take your depression seriously, and get help as soon as possible. It is important to know that a doctor can give you the talk therapy, and the medicines you need to treat depression. Your job is to admit to yourself that you are in trouble, and that you need help.

There are some common depression signs you need to look out for. Keep a notebook and write down your behavior and feelings. One of the signs is a loss of interest in the things you use to love doing. You may experience feeling of not caring anymore about things like cooking, cleaning, and other daily chores.

Pay attention to your appetite and weight. Check if anything changed lately. Some people will eat less, and lose weight when they are depressed. Others will eat more and gain weight. This is because everybody reacts differently to suffering and pain. The important thing is to notice if there is any big changes in your daily life.

Your sleep routine is also something to lookout for. Just like with eating, some people will sleep less while others will sleep almost all day long. Irritability is also another sign of depression. You may also feel like self-loathing, helplessness, or hopelessness. Loss of energy can also indicate a form of depression. If you have one or more of these symptoms, call your doctor today.

Chapter 2

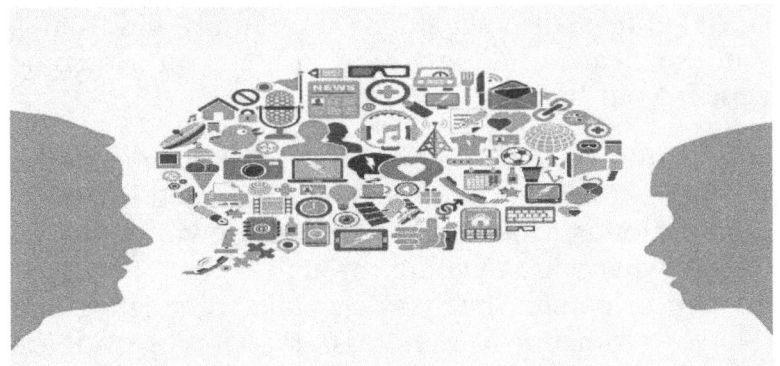

COMMUNICATE WITH FAMILY AND FRIENDS

Do not be ashamed to ask for help from the people around you. You are not the first, and unfortunately not the last to go through this. This is just like any other disease. Think of all the people who love you, and how much pain it would cause them if anything bad ever happened to you. To spare them this pain, communicate with them; don't be afraid to share all your dark thoughts. You don't need their opinion. A hug is sometimes enough. Saying things out loud can be like a wakeup call for you too. It can make you realize the gravity of the situation.

When you keep your thoughts to yourself, you can end up believing they are perfectly normal. When you communicate them to someone who cares you will feel much better. Why would you carry that amount of pain by yourself when there is someone who can share your burden? Do not think by telling them you are causing them distress. This is only temporary, and it's for the greater good. Imagine the horrible alternative. If something were to happen to you, they would blame themselves forever. So you are actually doing them a favor by telling them now. This will give them a chance to do everything in their power to save you from your thoughts. If you think about it, letting them know that you are thinking about suicide is not a selfish act at all. Your family and friends love you and they want to do anything to help you overcome this dark time in your life.

If you are not comfortable talking in front of everyone, choose one or two people. Make sure those people are good listeners. Another good option is to write your feelings down. This way you can express what you are going through better. You need to communicate in person, but you can take your letter and read it out loud to someone as well. Also read it when you are by yourself. Sometimes hearing yourself can make you understand your condition better. Ask yourself what you would advice a person going through the same thing that you are now. Learn how to become your own best friend. This doesn't mean you don't need anyone else in your life. Of course you do, but first of all you need to love yourself. By doing this you can protect yourself, and in the end this will make your family and friends happy.

Chapter 3

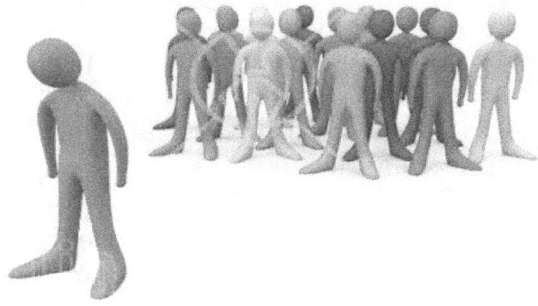

AVOID BEING ALONE

If you are depressed and have suicidal thoughts, most of the time you will prefer to be alone. However, social withdrawal in this situation can be very dangerous. You need to surround yourself with as many people as possible. This will not only distract you and help you get over those thoughts, but you will also have people to help you in case you lose control. The worst mistake you can make is thinking you cannot lose control, and nothing bad can happen.

Most suicidal thoughts are just thoughts, but some of them end in tragedy. To avoid being that small unfortunate percentage, try to prevent it by not being alone. If you live alone, ask a friend to move in for a couple of days. You can also move back home with your parents until you start feeling better. You will enjoy being their baby again, and allowing them to protect you from all the bad things in the world. Parents are on this earth for this, to take care of their children, and protect them from their self.

If someone you know is throwing a party do not decline the invitation. Go even if you don't feel like it. The worst thing that could happen is you will end up sitting down and watching other people have fun. This will give you some distraction, and also make sure you don't drink. Alcohol is not recommended in cases of depression, because it can worsen the symptoms.

If you are lucky to have a family, do not push them away. Your wife or husband only wants to help. Being around children can be beneficial as well. Borrow from their happiness, and learn how to be a careless child again. Organize a family camping trip. There is almost nothing better for you than being surrounded by nature with the people you love the most. Ask everyone to leave their electronic devices at home.

Chapter 4

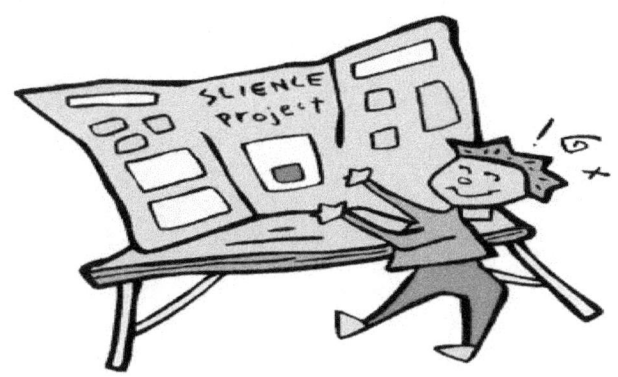

FIND NEW PROJECTS

The best cure for getting over any negative thoughts and suffering is to occupy your mind with something else. Find new projects, and keep yourself busy. Fill your day with all kind of things. This will make you feel useful, and it will give you purpose. You will be surprised to see how therapeutic work is. The best thing is that you don't have to pay for this kind of therapy. You are actually getting paid. Of course you can get involved in nonprofit projects too. For example charity works because when you help others you cannot put a price on it. The joy of making other people happy is priceless. Helping people in need is an excellent method to get over your own pain.

Search for a new job too. If you are already working, try to find something part time. This will give you no time for suicidal thoughts. At the end of a long day of work you will look forward to a nice dinner, and a good night sleep. The advantage of this approach is that you earn money too. This will allow you to splurge, and enjoy some luxury items you couldn't afford before. Life is made up of little pleasures. If you spend your time working hard and rewarding yourself, you will overcome depression, and dark thoughts on your own.

If you feel like you cannot handle it alone, you can also ask for help from your doctor.

Chapter 5

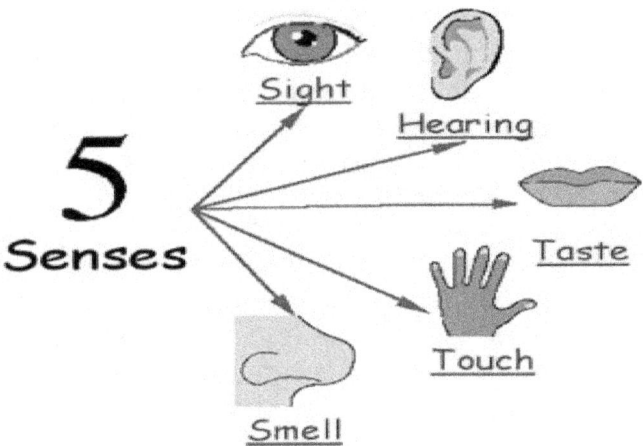

USE ALL OF YOUR SENSES

Use all your 5 senses to find some new coping resources. Try watching something soothing and nice. This can be anything from a painting, a movie, or just taking a walk to enjoy nature.

Take some time for yourself, and learn how to just relax. Don't think of anything. Leave the stress from work behind. Few people know that happiness is actually living in the moment.

Listen to some songs you love. Be careful not to listen to any songs that make you sad, or bring back bad memories. Music has a power over human beings. Use this to your advantage. You may have a few songs that put a smile on your face. Play them over and over until you feel that your mood is changing. You can also invite some friends over. You do not need to organize a party. Just get some snacks, some board games, and good music. This is all you need to feel better.

The sense of smell can also be used to overcome suicidal thoughts. Some smells can help you remember some good things in your pass, such as when you were a child and your mom was preparing your favorite dinner. Another example is a smell of perfume that can reminds you of your first love. Aroma therapy is another thing you can try. There are plenty of spa salons that offer the service. By smelling things you love you can change your mood and attitude.

Taste is also important. Savor all the food that you eat. Do not eat to stop feeling hunger. Choose foods that will bring back happy memories, and put you in a good mood. While you are going through a dark period, try to eat only your favorite foods. Do your best to choose the healthier options.

You can also use your sense of touch to find comfort, and help cope with any dark thoughts. Make sure you choose comfortable clothes to wear around the house. If you have a dog, spend some time petting him. This can also be done with a cat, or a horse. These pets are being used for soothing a lot of people who suffer from different types of mental and physical pain. There is something extremely comforting in the unconditional love you get from your pet. Getting a relaxing massage is another thing you can do. Take advantage of all your senses to make yourself feel good.

Chapter 6

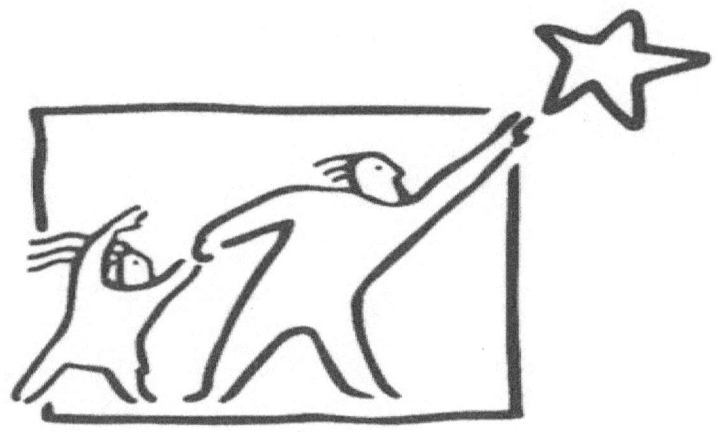

FIND NEW GOALS AND DREAMS FOR THE FUTURE

Always look towards the future. Do this with hope and optimism. Make a list of your dreams for the next year. What would you like to achieve? This can include material things,

but don't stop at that. You can also write down everything you want for your personal life. Write down the five most important goals for yourself, and put the list somewhere where you can see it. Whenever you have dark suicidal thoughts, look at that list. Will you want to miss all those amazing things? One or maybe all of them might just be around the corner. If your personal life is the main problem, try to focus on your career for now. Things will get better when you least expect it.

If your career is the problem, take a vacation, and enjoy it with your family. Sometimes taking a break from what causes you stress is beneficial. When you go back to work you will have new strength to fight.

As soon as you achieve one goal, take some time off to congratulate yourself. The next step is to start focusing on the next thing you want. This is the way to keep looking towards tomorrow, and staying positive. Also, remember that life is full of surprises. Things don't always go as planned. Do not regard this as a negative or a failure. This is part of the excitement of life. If we always get what we want, when we want it, life would be very boring.

Chapter 7

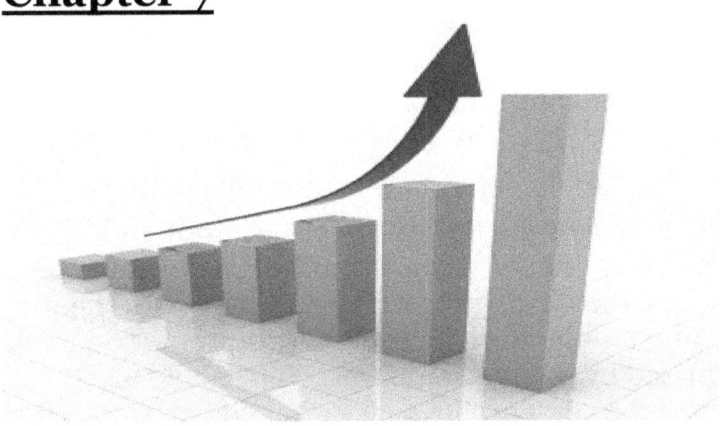

BREAK YOUR EXPECTATION INTO PARTS

Most people get depressed when they don't achieve all their goals. Take a better look at the things that you want. Maybe it's time to lower your expectations (just a little). If you have a good goal to achieve, try to break it into parts. This way, every step you succeed to achieve, is a small victory. By doing this, you avoid disappointment and depression. Give yourself more time to obtain all you want in life.

When you expect too much from yourself, you might end up feeling worthless. This is an easy trap to fall into. Be smart about it, and avoid it by celebrating every little success you have. Remember that each step you make is a step closer towards what you want to obtain.

For example, you may be suffering because all your friends are married and you are still single, imagine that special someone is around the corner, waiting for you. You might meet him or her tomorrow. Age doesn't matter at all. Love and happiness come when you least expect it. In situations like this, people tend to avoid their married friends. This is a mistake because you need to learn how to accept the reality of your life. There is nothing wrong with being single, and it doesn't mean you will be that way forever.

Another example is having high expectations from your job. You are working really hard, and instead of being promoted, your boss acts like you don't exist. The solution for this is to start searching for a new job, or just try to be happy with the position you currently have. If the last option is not something you want, set up a meeting with your boss. Share with them how you feel, and tell them why you deserve a promotion. You might be surprised by his or her answer. You should also consider that maybe you are so good at what you do your boss cannot find a replacement as good as you. Whatever the case, always try to see the good side of things.

Chapter 8

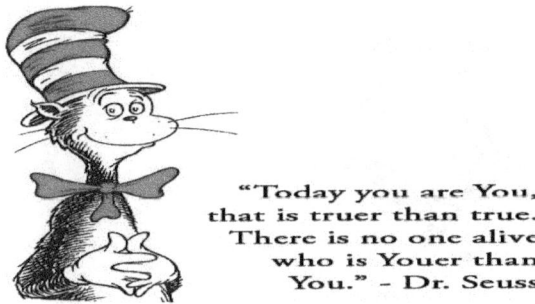

"Today you are You,
that is truer than true.
There is no one alive
who is Youer than
You." - Dr. Seuss

POSITIVE AFFIRMATIONS

Life is worth living, and you need to convince yourself of this.
An efficient way to do this is by using positive affirmations.
Just like everything else in life, depression, disappointments,
and suicidal thoughts are all temporary. The way you feel
today will change tomorrow. Repeat these words to yourself
until you start seeing positive changes. You can also say that
you are strong, and nothing can break your spirit. The key to
positive affirmations is to actually believe them. Train your
brain into believing that you are an amazing person who can
succeed anything in life. This is not a lie. If you believe in
yourself, and learn how to be positive, there is nothing you
cannot do.

There are plenty of positive affirmations you can use, but you
should create your own. Each person is different, and you
know best what works for you. The affirmations are in fact
words of encouragement that you repeat to yourself. You
make this a routine until you feel that you are stronger, and
believe in yourself. It is important to repeat the affirmations
out loud. When you repeat affirmations out loud your brain

will perceive them as an order that need to be obeyed.

Chapter 9

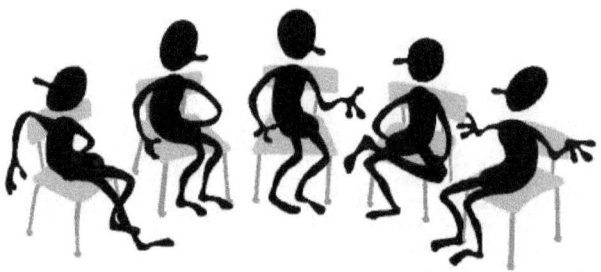

GO TO THERAPY

You can get rid of suicidal thoughts by yourself, but just to be safe, always go to therapy as well. A professional will be able to diagnose your health problem, and tell you what needs to be done. There are plenty of doctors or therapist to choose from. It is important to pick one you feel comfortable with. Interview them before you choose one. This person will be the one hearing all your intimate thoughts. If for any reason you don't trust your doctor or therapist, move on to the next one. Just like you would do with any type of relationship, it has to have that special chemistry.

During therapy, don't be scared to ask all the questions you have on your list. The doctor is there to help you. Consider the room your safety place. As you probably know, you have doctor-patient confidentiality, and anything you say will stay between the two of you. Therefore, there is no need to feel scared or ashamed. Let it all out, and leave each therapy session feeling lighter and stronger. The doctor or therapist will teach you how to cope with stress and depression. They will also give you the right tools to overcome suicidal thoughts. Do not postpone going to therapy because it is a matter of life and death. Most people feel they can do it all on their own, but it is always safer to have the confirmation from a professional.

Therapy can last as long as your doctor thinks it is necessary. You need to have patience, and not end it sooner than the doctor recommends. Clear your schedule and make your therapy a priority. If you had a physical life threatening disease you would seek help right away. Imagine this is the same situation. Depression and suicidal thoughts are just as serious as any other disease. Many people are embarrassed to admit they go to therapy. They think that people will judge them, and they prefer not go at all.

This is the wrong way to look at it, and if you are one of those people, try to change your mentality. Therapy is not just for people with mental illnesses. You can go through a difficult period in your life, and need a few sessions. Therapy is the way to treat depression, and get over a trauma from your present or past. This is also the way to get over the suicidal thoughts, and help put you on the road to recovery.

Conclusion

Thank you again for choosing this book!

I hope this book was able to give you the confidents you need to reduce, and eventually eliminate suicidal thoughts.

According to statistics, 90% of the people who have suicidal thoughts manage to overcome them. Unfortunately, 10% end up putting their dark thoughts into practice. The good news is that you can avoid this by recognizing you need help to change the way you are thinking. As soon as you realize that you have a problem, ask for help. Surround yourself with friends and family, and try to keep busy.

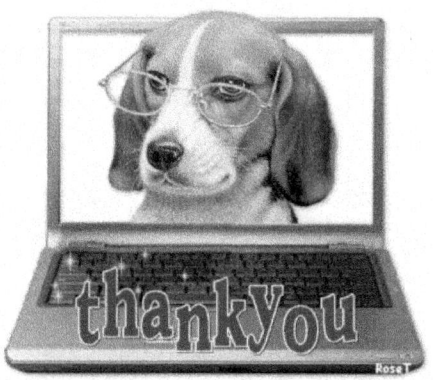

Finally, if you enjoyed this book, would you be kind enough to leave a review for this book on Amazon? It'd be greatly appreciated!

Thank you and good luck!

Preview Of 'THE DEPRESSION CURE: How to Overcome Depression and become Depression Free'

CHAPTER 1: MOOD DISORDER
Tackling depression head-on the right way

Recovery begins when we overcome depression and become totally depression free. Treatment for depression starts when one recognizes the symptoms and began to seek help. To find a Depression cure it requires patience from both the individual and the physician. Depression is not like normal sadness and happiness if you are experiencing feelings of despair, or hopelessness. Most people do not realize they are depressed and let this illness go unnoticed.

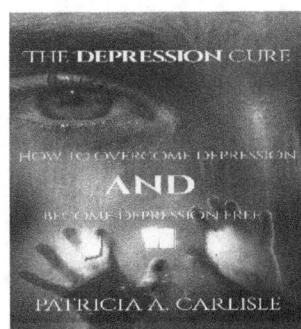

THE DEPRESSION CURE: How to overcome depression and become depression free.

Check Out My Other Books

Below you'll find some of my other popular books that are popular on Amazon and Kindle as well. Alternatively, you can visit my author page on Amazon to see other work done by me. (https://amazon.com/author/patriciacarlisle)

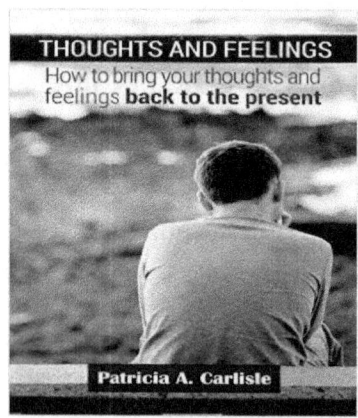

THOUGHTS AND FEELINGS: How to bring your thoughts and feelings back to the present.

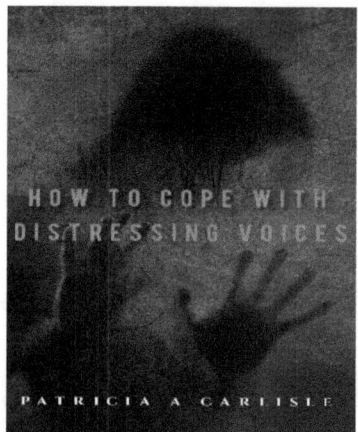

HOW TO COPE WITH DISTRESSING VOICES.

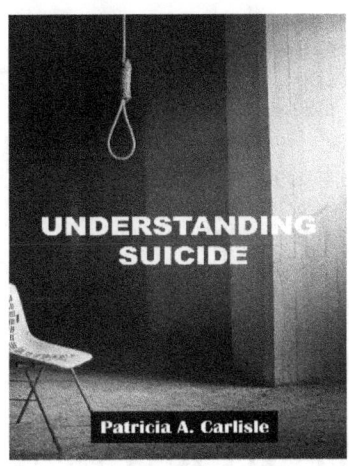

UNDERSTANDING SUICIDE.

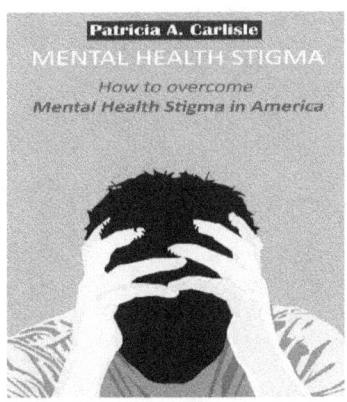

MENTAL HEALTH STIGMA: How to overcome Mental Health Stigma in America.

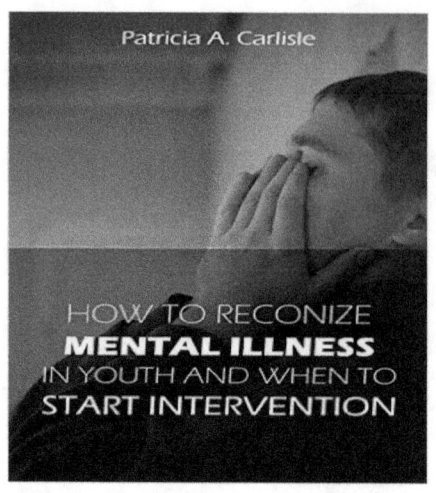

HOW TO RECOGNIZE MENTAL ILLNESS IN YOUTH:
and when to Start Intervention.

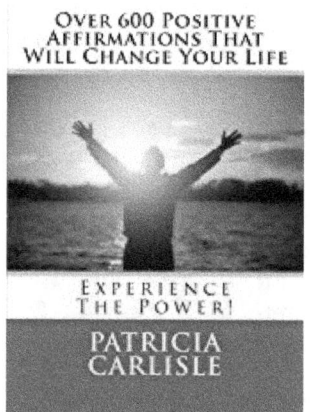

OVER 600 POSITIVE AFFIRMATIONS THAT WILL
CHANGE YOUR LIFE. EXPERIENCE THE POWER!

BONUS: SUBSCRIBE TO THE FREE BOOK

Beginners Guide to Yoga & Meditation

"Stressed out? Do You Feel Like The World Is Crashing Down Around You? Want To Take A Vacation That Will Relax Your Mind, Body And Spirit? Well this Easy To Read Step By Step

E-Book Makes It All Possible!"

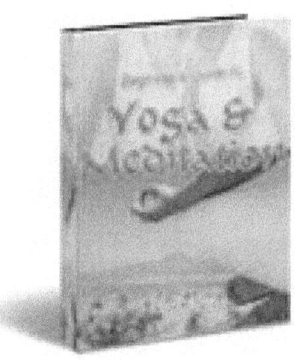

Instructions on how to join our mailing list, and receive a free copy of "Yoga and Meditation" can be found in any of my Kindle eBooks.

NOTES

NOTES

NOTES

NOTES

NOTES

NOTES

www.ingramcontent.com/pod-product-compliance
Lightning Source LLC
Chambersburg PA
CBHW070751180526
45168CB00004B/1585